A Simple Guide to Natural Healing for Everyone

by a Practising Healer

HAROLD KING

authorHOUSE®

AuthorHouse™ UK Ltd.
500 Avebury Boulevard
Central Milton Keynes, MK9 2BE
www.authorhouse.co.uk
Phone: 08001974150

First published by AuthorHouse 3/6/2008

ISBN: 978-1-4343-7129-4 (sc)

Printed in the United States of America
Bloomington, Indiana
This book is printed on acid-free paper.

NOTE: *The Code of Conduct does not preclude a Healer from giving First Aid to a human or an animal, in an emergency, without querying Doctor's or Veterinary Surgeon's involvement. In this case the Healer is attempting to preserve life, prevent further injury and/or aid recovery.*

ACKNOWLEDGEMENTS

I would like to thank the following for their help and inspiration.

My wife, who instigated the book, telling me to get on with it in her gentle way (I've still got the scars to prove it).

My Healing colleagues, students, past and present, who, possibly unknowingly, have made their contribution.

Last, but not least, Dean Shah. Publishing Advisor and the AuthorHouse team, for their sincere help and encouragement.

CONTENTS

FOREWORD

This book is written to try to give a more modern view of Natural or Spiritual Healing. Healing is now subject to many more Regulations and a true Practising Healer is bound by a strict Code of Conduct which is often referred to in the following. It is an attempt to remove any mystique and to accept Healing as a natural process.

It must be emphasised that these are my own thoughts and apply to Natural or Spiritual Healing, not to any other therapy.

Since commencing this book, I understand that a change in Government Regulations is proposed for April, 2008. These rules would make strict adherence to the present training and Code of Conduct of paramount importance. Although Natural or Spiritual Healing is a 'Complimentary' therapy and completely non-invasive the training requires more dedication and commitment than many 'Alternative' therapies, which could be termed invasive.

CHAPTER ONE

HISTORY OF HEALING

Healing has been practised for thousands of years in many countries and communities. We can find proof of Spiritual Healing going back 15,000 years to the caveman. Caves in Central and Western France show a remarkable display of painted hands, depicting healing images.

Shamanic traditions, which are as old as mankind, acknowledge all of mankind, the physical, mental, emotional and spiritual. Their concept of health was based on people being in harmony. Chinese medicine dates back about 5,000 years. In the olden times religion and healing went together. The origin of medicine was regarded as magic – anything beyond the normal was regarded as magic. About 500 B.C. the Greeks introduced Hygienic Therapy, which is rest, fresh air and diet as principal weapons against disease. We come forward to about 400 B.C. for

Hippocrates, who is regarded as the father of medicine. He played an important part in laying the foundations of scientific medicine and separating it from speculation and superstition. The Hippocratic Oath represents his ethical position. Here is a rough translation from a passage he wrote – "It is believed by experienced doctors that the heat that oozes from the hand, on being applied to the sick, is highly salutary. It has often appeared, while I have been soothing my patients, as if there is a

singular property in my hands to pull and draw away from the affected parts aches and diverse impurities, by laying my hands upon that place".

Coming to more modern times – Jesus said to his disciples, "Go forth and heal".

From about 350 A.D. people went to the Church for healing. This was seen as absolution.

In some cultures the practice in intercession for healing with Mankind's Spiritual Force has been and still is the prerogative of selected people, king, priest, rabbi, monk, elder, prophet, witch doctor and so on, who are acknowledged to have a talent for healing. In Britain during the reign of the Stuarts and Tudors the 'Royal Touch' was very popular. After prayer the King would touch the sufferer with his hand and then give him a coin. The practice of Royal Healing reached its' peak at the end of the Seventeenth Century when Charles 2nd was giving the Royal Touch to around 5,000 sufferers a year. Even into the nineteen hundreds other healers were regarded as witches and could be arrested for intercession.

It is now recognised that healing is more widespread than previously understood. Throughout the world many people are dedicated to helping others, using healing through prayer or by the laying on of hands, as an active part of their philosophy of life and religious practice, whatever that may be...

Nowadays a growing number of doctors refer their patients to Healers or have them working in their practices. Healers also work in hospitals, nursing homes and hospices.

CHAPTER TWO

WHAT IS HEALING

Healing is normally referred to as Spiritual or Natural Healing in an attempt to describe its' source. A brief definition would be, "Transfer, via the Healer, of a natural energy source within the Universe". Natural Healing is non-religious and universal, in that it encompasses all faiths and non-believers. The object of healing is to restore balance within the body and create harmony of mind, body and spirit. To relax and calm the patient to give time and space for the immune system to work. We all know that there is a built-in power of self healing which we call our immune system. Without it we would succumb to any virus or infection if not given outside help. With any power there has to be a source from which this power ensues. Depending on a person's beliefs this power is given different names, but no one denies its' existence.

Many theories, most of which raise more questions than answers, have been suggested as to why and how healing works. We know it does work, so do the whys and wherefores really matter? There are many mysteries in the world, not everything is fully understood, but some are accepted. We place a seed in the ground and it grows, there small seeds can grow into mighty trees. Not many of us stop to think why this happens to that seed, it is accepted as a 'natural process'. Does healing plant the seed that activates a person's immune system thereby starting the 'healing process'?

The following quote is from the April,2007, issue of the Reader's Digest Magazine:- "While no one can actually prove that prayer can cure illness, many doctors cite cases of recovery that cannot be attributed to any other reason. What we do know is that religion and spirituality can reduce stress and boost the immune system.

"Population studies have shown that those who regularly go to church live on average seven years longer than those who aren't religious", says Anne Douglas, chair of Scotland's Christian Fellowship of Healing. Several studies have looked at spirituality and the immune function and found a connection.

In a 1997 study of older adults by Dr. Harold Koenig, Professor of Psychiatry and Behavioural Sciences said that – people who attend religious services had a far healthier immune system than those who did not attend. A study in 2001 of women with metastatic breast cancer found that women who rated spirituality as important had a greater number of circulating white blood cells and total lymphocyte counts- reflecting stronger immune systems – than those who did not.

A 2002 study of Aids patients found that the most religious patients had the lowest levels of stress hormone cortisol and that the frequency of prayer was significantly related to longer survival".

The more we think about this article, the greater the connection with Spiritual or Natural Healing. The people mentioned are obviously all connecting by prayer to some Natural Energy Source and benefiting from that connection. In Healing the connection is made, possibly more strongly because of a set purpose, to the source through attunement. Attunement is explained later. The purpose is to create harmony of mind, body and spirit to help the immune system of the patient. As can be seen by this article the connection results in a far healthier immune system by increasing the lymphocyte count. It would follow that Natural or Spiritual Healing creates a form of leucocytosis increasing the number of white blood cells in the lymph nodes to fight any form of disease.

Use of the hands to convey healing had been practised for many years as previously stated. This is a natural reaction used by us all, even as a child. Remember when we suffer physical hurt it is an unconscious and natural reaction to rub the area involved, we first did this as a child.

Healing can take many forms, some of which may not be realised when applied, but still exist. A child upset or frightened will run to mother for comfort, this is a form of healing. Anyone troubled or upset for any reason

and has counselling is receiving healing.. These are all non-invasive as is Natural or Spiritual Healing, nothing is applied or taken. Therefore Healing should not be referred to as an Alternative Therapy, but as Complimentary being complementary to Allopathic Medicine.

Music plays an important role in healing. At most healing sessions quiet background music is played. The music played is meditative and soothing helping the Patient/client to relax. As previously stated that aim of healing is to create harmony of mind, body and spirit. Music is the harmony of sound, rhyme is the harmony of words. Combine music and rhyme and we arrive at the Music of Healing:

Songs of today and tomorrow
And of the future to come
These are the things we can borrow
Then to the music succumb
Singing can lift up your spirits
And it can lighten your heart
Help you to dump all your troubles
Into nature's dustcart
When you are feeling downhearted
And every world trouble is yours
Listen to all of life's music
And worries seep out of your pores
When you are passing on healing
And you feel your confidence fall
Music can lift up your feelings
That's part of God's gift to us all.

Think more deeply of harmony in all things. When all parts are in harmony, machinery works more efficiently and smoothly. We look at beautiful landscapes and vistas and we see nature in harmony. If only nations could work in harmony we could achieve world peace and many more benefits would naturally follow. This is all part of healing working naturally to heal the world and heal each other.

CHAPTER 3

THE HEALER AND TRAINING

How to describe a Healer? Adult – male or female. Age – immaterial. Shape – any as long as breathing and reasonably active. Disposition – kind, generous, non-judgemental and compassionate with a desire to help others. Intelligence – reasonable with the ability to understand requirements appertaining to healing. As can be seen this applies to most people, so anyone fitting the foregoing can become a Healer with the appropriate training.

A true Natural Healer does not rely on gimmicks. He/she does not wave arms about and make extravagant gestures over the patient/client to try to impress. Healing does not require these gestures as they have no value in healing and can hold the procedure up to ridicule.

Training takes place, as a student healer, over a period of two years under the supervision of a Full Healer, who needs to hold a Certificate as a Tutor. The Full Healer will be a member of an Approved Healing Association. Meaning approved by the Confederation of Healing Organisations. Currently the Spiritual or Natural Healing Organisations are self-regulated. The Healing Organisations work together under advice from the Foundation for Integrated Medicine to establish good standards of healing practice. The training over this two year period will require knowledge of healing practices and procedures. Some knowledge of physiology and anatomy, basic first aid, nature of disease, listening skills, attunement, meditation, visualisation, record keeping – together with security and confidentiality, some awareness of the various laws that affect relationship between Healer and client. Familiarisation with the Code of Conduct to which all Approved Healing Associations must comply. This may seem a formidable task at first glance, but remember this is over a period of two years with generally weekly practice of two hour meetings, with many instances of practical healing sessions and revision. One of the most important parts is knowledge of the Code of Conduct which must be strictly adhered to for the protection of both the Healer and the client. Attunement is harmony of mind, body and spirit, acquired through practice. When fully attuned with connection to the natural energy source the Healer feels this connection. This may be felt in different ways. Some may feel warmth or pressure around the crown of the head, others pressure in the centre of the forehead, others warmth around the heart, still others tingling in the hands and fingers. There could just be one or a combination of these feelings.

On joining an Approved Healing Association the student is issued with a Probationer's Membership Card and is covered by Personal Liability Insurance, an important requirement. At the end of the, at least, two year period, the student is assessed by an Independent Assessor. The Probationer's Card is changed to Full after successfully completing training and assessment. When healing, this card should be produced, on demand, as proof of identity and insurance. This is also a safeguard to assure the patient/client that the Healer has been properly trained and is working in accordance with the Code of Conduct. It is advisable for a prospective client to ask to see this card for their own protection.

CHAPTER 4

MEET THE HEALER
CONTACT AND DISTANT HEALING

When first meeting a patient or client, the initial contact is important as this can influence the whole healing session. The Healer's approach should be such as to inspire confidence and put the patient at ease. The procedure should be explained and the patient given the opportunity to give any relevant information and a record should be made of any relevant details. This, of course, would not be necessary at a demonstration or a one-off session where there is unlikely to be any repeat sessions. The patient/client must be given the chance to see the information entered and correct if necessary. Permission must always be requested before commencing contact healing, with the assurance that the hands will not be placed anywhere likely to cause embarrassment.

The Healer must comply with the Code of Conduct. He must not give massage, clairvoyant messages or suggest the taking of medicines of any kind. The Healer must never remove or re-arrange the patient's clothing.

This does not prohibit the patient from removing outer garments for comfort. The Healer must never interfere with any instructions given by the patient's doctor.

During the healing session the patient/client may feel heat or cold from the Healer's hands or may feel a tingling sensation. The more relaxed the patient can be the more benefit they are likely to derive from the healing and the more they are likely to experience. Patients often sense the presence of others and often feel as though other hands have been placed upon them. Overall there is nearly always a feeling of peace and the calming of the mind and body. Just occasionally the patient may not feel much at the time, but will get a good night's sleep and feel better the next day. It is most unusual for the patient not to feel anything. With a patient who is suffering from physical pain, at the time of the healing session, this pain sometimes temporarily increases, before fading. The Healer may not always place a hand over the area where the patient has indicated that there is discomfort. A pain may be caused by some dysfunction in another area. Healing goes to where it is required. It is not directed by the Healer, but more by the patient's own immune system. It must be remembered that the Healer is merely a channel for the Healing Power and does not, personally, control the healing. The object of the healing session is to try to achieve the balance of mind, body and spirit, so to activate the immune system to correct any imbalance that may be the cause of the patient's disquiet or ailment. As a Healer I always like to regard the session as "healing with the patient" rather that "to the patient". Giving healing to the patient suggests that the Healer is personally doing something to the patient. Whereas, to repeat the true state, the Healer is merely a channel.

The more the patient and the Healer can become attuned to each other, the more powerful the healing can be. When this takes place, the patient will often have a feeling of peace and calm, the breathing will slow down, giving the body time to rest and heal. It must be realised that no one can get rid of something that they subconsciously want to keep. Just occasionally a person can, subconsciously, be relying on an ailment to give them an excuse not to perform some task. Especially if the task is one they do not like.

After the healing session the Healer must make sure that the patient is fully aware of their surroundings, as occasionally a patient may feel slightly drowsy or confused after being totally relaxed. The session should be discussed and any reactions noted in the patient's presence, so completing the records of the healing session. (Once again, if at a clinic or regular healing session) All records are strictly confidential and must be kept secure, as stated in CHAPTER 3.

We now come to Distant Healing, sometimes referred to as Absent Healing. Distant Healing would appear to be a more correct description, as the healing is not absent, the only thing absent is the physical presence of the patient at the healing session. Distant Healing can be sent in response to a letter or telephone call or by verbal request. When Distant Healing is sent in reply to any request, then the Healer's healing thoughts are centred on the person only. Some very good results are achieved from the method.

Distant Healing can be more effective if the Healer can visualise the person concerned smiling and clear of the reason for the request for healing.

At training sessions, with students, a short Distant Healing session is often held, where group healing thoughts can be directed to any individual, or transmitted to form a reservoir from which anyone crying out for help can draw in their hour of need, like turning on the tap and drawing water.

CHAPTER 5

REFLECTIONS ON CHAKRAS
AND THE AURA

This CHAPTER may appear controversial in view of past writings, but I am not attempting to deny the existence of Chakras or the Aura. The attempt is to take a different view, which is more easily acceptable to a down-to-earth practical person. Trying to remove any air of mystique or magic, thoughts giving a more modern explanation.

The earliest mention of the word 'Chakra' is said to come from the Vedas, the four holy books of the Hindus, believed to date back to before 2,500 B.C. Certain parts of the body were found to be centres of energy – there is no argument about this. All credit is due to whoever made this discovery all those thousands of years ago.

This knowledge was acquired long before the power of electricity was known and recognised. Medical science has advanced and we know that the position of the major chakras coincide with the main endocrine glands and the nerve centres.

Now we think of the body's nervous system and think of the messages pulsing out from the brain. Compare this to the electrical wiring system of a house. This has a system of main junctions boxes (endocrine glands) and minor junction boxes (minor glands and lymph glands). These are needed to power all lights and appliances. The body is similar with the ganglia of nerves dividing and sub-dividing at different parts of the body.

It follows that the larger the junction box the more energy emanating from that position, as with the endocrine glands. The pulsing would obviously result from the passing of messages from the brain and also from the fact that all parts of the body are fed with life giving blood by the pulsing of the heart.

So are the main chakras the ancient name for the endocrine glands (the main junction boxes) and the minor chakras corresponding to the minor glands and lymph glands (the minor junction boxes)? Is the name still being used to create an air of mystique? No one is trying to deny the existence of these areas of energy, merely applying a more modern view.

Now we come to the Aura. Once again the existence of the Aura has been accepted for thousands of years as a subtle energy field around the body. We now know that this is an electromagnetic field which surrounds the physical body. Such a field surrounds power lines, pylons and mobile phone masts.

This field around the body is not visible to normal vision, but some people have the ability (either natural or developed) to see the energy field.

It appears as a white smoky haze, similar to a heat haze, or to the more sensitive observer, as a radiance of moving, swirling colours. It can be felt or sensed by various dousing methods. Kirlian photography (a Russian invention) can capture this bio-electric energy on film, producing Polaroid colour photographs.

Can we analyse this field to make it more understandable to everyone?

We understand it as an energy field emitted from the passage of energies passing through the human body. As such it can be said to be a reflection of the bodily activities, which if not working correctly (as a broken fuse) must show up some defect in the area where the malfunction occurs, as with chakras.

Here we come to the area of mystique or magic instilled into dealing with auras and chakras. The healing and cleansing of auras and chakras. The question is;- can one heal a reflection? When a woman looks at her reflection in the mirror and sees her lips are pale, where does she apply the lipstick? Obviously on the lips and this cures the reflection. It is said that even when a limb is amputated, the aura still remains around the area. In this case that part of the aura must show some defect. The only way this defect could be eliminated would be to remove the cause, in other words re-grow the limb by healing the aura. To my knowledge this has never been accomplished.

Logically it must be the same with all defects shown in the energy reflection or aura. Some believe that the aura remaining around the amputated limb is the reason why pain or itching is sometimes felt as though coming from the missing limb. A more logical and scientific explanation is that the nerve endings in the brain can live on, even for years, after the amputation.

So what conclusion can we draw from this? It would appear that waving the hands about over the body cannot really achieve anything because this is simply trying to work on a reflection with both chakras and the aura. Shaking the hands to remove toxins after passing the hands over the body would seem to be for demonstrations purposes only and could result in bringing ridicule on the healing purpose. The healing intention may be good, but we must think of the possible impressions given to a critical observer.

The only answer would appear to be in the healing of the cause of the defect so that the reflection would then be clear of malfunction, as there is then no malfunction to reflect.

The colour, observed by some, emanating from these energy centres or from the energy waves around the body; would be that these energy waves are refractive and reflect colours when exposed to light. Differentials in these energy waves would be caused by malfunctions in the organs emitting these waves.

We now consider the seven layers of the Aura and their colours, the seven colours of the rainbow corresponding to the colours given to the main Chakras, red, orange, yellow, etc., in that order. Place a piece of cut glass, or a polished crystal, in the sunlight and see the reflections cast onto a plain surface. We get the colours of the rainbow, in layers, each layer interpenetrating the layer below as the Aura is seen or photographed. The Aura is described as a subtle energy field, therefore has not got the refractive power of the solid cut glass or crystal. This would account for the Aura and its' colours only being visible to some and not to all observers.

With Natural Healing we know that the healing goes to where it is required, therefore there is no need for the Healer to direct it to any particular point. In any case this would be ' ego healing ' and could interfere with the healing energies. To say that there was some defect in a chakra or in the aura, indicating a malfunction in a certain area, would be a form of diagnosis, strictly forbidden by the Code of Conduct. It appears that the only way to achieve maximum benefit from healing is to perform the act in accordance with the methods stated in the previous CHAPTERs and strictly in accordance with our Code of Conduct.

CHAPTER 6

SELF-HEALING, VISUALISATION, AND MEDITATION

Self-healing, Visualisation and Meditation are all inter-connected, as all can be used to achieve the similar result. As with Natural Healing these exercises are completely non-religious and can be practised by everyone.

We think of the body, to some degree, as a machine. All machines are not built perfectly, as we know, some are produced with defects. With the body, modern medical science can work on the D.N.A. and remove certain defects before they have the chance to develop. Then throughout life we are not totally immune to various diseases and viruses, therefore we need help to overcome these. In many cases it is necessary to seek the help of the doctor, but even in these events it is possible to aid the recovery by self-healing, visualisation or meditation. With lesser ailments our own immune system can fight the disharmony in an effective manner, once again we can speed the recovery by creating a positive attitude. Might be thought of as "mind over matter".

Here we have the connection between self-healing and visualisation.

When we are feeling off-colour or ill, we all know which part of the body is suffering. There is some similarity between self-healing and distant healing, as the procedure is somewhat similar. We have to think of the part of the body where the discomfort lies. This is where some knowledge of anatomy can help, because if you know what organ, tissue, muscle or bone is in that area, it is easier to visualise. Now we concentrate our mind on the affected area and instead of being angry or annoyed with the malfunction. We think of it with love and see it glowing with health, with all pain removed. This may be a little difficult at first. But becomes easier with practice. Remember love makes the world go round. We are creating a positive frame of mind to aid and strengthen our immune system.

A second, slightly more complicated, visualisation which often works better with some is as follows. As with most things the appeal depends on a person's mind set and possibly on their metabolism.

Here we visualise ourselves totally enclosed in a large egg. We use the egg shape as it symbolises the beginning of life. We are totally enclosed and protected within this cocoon. We visualise ourselves seated comfortably in a chair, fully relaxed. We don't necessarily have to be alone, we can have a favourite companion with us if this gives more peace of mind. The walls of the shell around us have many shelves, on these shelves are medicines and tablets of every kind. As we concentrate and visualise our pain and discomfort, as in the previous visualisation, we are drawn to the appropriate medicine or tablets, to cure the affliction. We then see and feel the pain and discomfort fading as the medicine takes effect.

Of course, we are not always ill and there are ways to help to give ourselves protection and to strengthen the immune system to help alleviate the dangers of being susceptible to viruses and infections.

One is a Body Awareness Exercise that can be combined with expanding the electromagnetic field (the aura) around the body. For this exercise you must find time and space where you are unlikely to be disturbed. When first attempting this exercise it can take a few minutes, but with practice the time can be drastically reduced.

Sit comfortably in an upright chair, spine as straight as possible, feet uncrossed and flat on the floor. Some may prefer to sit cross-legged on a cushion, with palms facing up, linking thumb and first finger together. As a beginner the first position is easier and more comfortable.

Close your eyes and take a few deep breaths down into the abdomen. At the same time feeling yourself relax from head to toe. Become aware of your toes and feet, allowing them to relax and feeling warm and comfortable. Slowly move your concentration upwards through toes, feet and legs feeling each relax in turn. Continue moving your thoughts up through the body, focusing on each part in turn. Feel each part relax into harmony with the whole of the body.

When your concentration reaches the level of the eyes, pause and focus in the centre of the forehead. This is one of the main control centres of the body and can control and balance all body and mind activities. Try to bring your whole consciousness and concentration to this area and feel your whole body in harmony.

The exercise can be ended at this point by giving yourself a few moments before carrying on with your normal activities, or can be combined with the expanding of the aura.

To combine the Body Awareness with a Protection Exercise carry on as follows. When you bring your whole consciousness to bear on the centre of the forehead, continue your deeper breathing and imagine you are breathing out through this point in the centre of the forehead. At the same time imagine that your whole body is surrounded by a bubble of white or golden light. Your body is filled with this light. As you breath out you are expanding the bubble away from your body until you feel comfortable with the distance and protected within the bubble. With practice you can expand the auric protection shield around the body at any time, if you feel threatened or vulnerable. As before, on completion of this exercise, give yourself a few moments before carrying on with your normal activities.

There is also a short breathing exercise to help strengthen the auric field around the body.

As previously mentioned the electromagnetic field around the body is seen in seven layers. We can use this to our advantage in the balancing and strengthening of the aura. This exercise, being short, can be practised early in the morning, before going to bed each night and at any convenient time during the day.

Once again we think of the egg. Imagine yourself the yolk inside the egg, between yourself and the shell are seven other layers, representing the seven layers of the aura. We begin taking good, deep breaths, trying to take the same time over the in-breath and with the out-breath. On the in-breath imagine you are breathing up the back of the body from the feet to the top of the head. On the out-breath breathe down the front of the body and under the feet, where the in-breath commenced, thereby completing the circle. The next in-breath is up the right hand side of the body- again from the feet – to the top of the head. The out-breath is down the left hand side of the body sweeping under the feet to form the complete circle.

Repeat each of these breaths seven times. Each time imagine that the circle is moving a little further away from the body. When you have completed seven breaths around the back and front of the body and seven breaths around the sides, you are sweeping in a much wider circle.

When we take the in-breaths we are breathing in peace and calm. On the out-breaths we are letting go of all tensions and worries. As can be seen this exercise can be completed in fourteen breaths.

Now we consider Meditation as a further method of bringing peace and calm to the mind, also balancing the mind and all bodily functions. The main difference between visualisation and meditation is that in visualisation the mind is active and full of thoughts, whereas, in meditation the aim is to empty the mind and still all active thought. This gives the body rest and space and time for the immune system to carry out possible repairs, creating an inner stillness to help cope with the pace of modern life.

Once again we need to find a quiet place, where we can be comfortable and unlikely to be disturbed. With this exercise we can sit in a chair, as in the body awareness exercise, with the head supported or, if preferred, try lying on the floor with the head on a cushion. Making sure we are warm and comfortable.

There are many ways to meditate, some are active in the beginning, but, as stated, this should lead to inaction and the emptying of the mind.

Passive: Allow thoughts to surface then drift away.

Mental: Concentrate the mind on a sphere of colour, preferably blue, lavender or violet.

Active: Count breaths up to ten, over and over, noting the air coming in and going out

Mantra: Choose a word of two or three syllables, with no real meaning, and keep repeating this. Or choose a word like peace or love and keep repeating this.

Imagining:-   Imagine a circular pool of still water. Any thoughts cause ripples on the water, mentally smooth away these ripples. Or, visualise a colour filling the whole of your inner view, as though inside behind the eyes, see this colour disappear into a dot. If thoughts start to rise again, repeat the process.

Complete relaxation may be difficult at first, but perseverance can pay dividends. Some people are lucky, choosing the right method for them and achieving the desired result quickly. Attempting to meditate after a heavy meal would generally be unsuccessful.

As in Natural and Distant Healing, music can play a very important part in Visualisation and Meditation. There are numerous cassettes and C.Ds where the music is specially formulated to create the right atmosphere for these exercises. Some of these are compiled totally of music, others contain the softly spoken words to lead you into a euphoric state to help with visualisation and meditation. A true visualisation would contain descriptive dialogue leading you to complete relaxation, where you would utilise all five senses in some way, before returning to full awareness of your surroundings. Meditation music flows and washes over you so that your mind concentrates on the music to remove all other thoughts from your mind, so that your body and mind are filled with peace and calm.

One element, so far not mentioned, that is important when passing on, or receiving healing is plain drinking water. I understand that water is the only fluid that is completely absorbed by the body. Hardly any of us drink enough plain water, which helps to flush away toxins and other impurities, which could be detrimental to general health. Especially after a healing session a glass of water should always be provided for both the healer and the patient, as both often feel the need.

Our general demeanour can have much to do with our general health and sense of well being. Anger, resentment and the inability to forgive and forget can have a detrimental effect on our enjoyment of life and our health. Look at anger and resentment, which are negative feelings and recognise them for what they are. Try to see a positive side in the situation and concentrate on that, in most cases the anger will fade. If we could all treat each other as we ourselves would like to be treated, this would be a marvellous beginning. We are all here with a purpose in life, but our true purpose is sometimes hard to see. Which brings us to this conclusion:-

This is no time to stand and stare
That's no way to see what's there
All the stress and all the strain
This everlasting pounding train
Of thoughts that flicker as they will
This is no time for standing still
We all are here to do our best
To live, to learn, to pass the test
We all must leave this mortal plain
But, first, must learn for why we came.

CHAPTER 7

FREQUENTLY ASKED QUESTIONS

How much will the healing cost?

Many Healers do not make any charge for healing. Most will accept a voluntary donation to help to cover any expenses. Many Healers have suffered some illness or pain in the past and recovered, possibly with some help from Natural Healing and are trying to give something back to help others. If attending a Clinic there should be a list of charges. It is always advisable to ask before a session starts.

How long will it take? How many sessions will I need?

A healing session usually takes 20 to 30 minutes. First session a little longer to take relevant information. The number of sessions can vary, often in accordance with the length of time the patient has had the trouble. One session can be sufficient in some cases. Many patients attend more often because they enjoy the experience. The decision is up to the patient.

What do I do and what will I feel?

Just relax and think of something you really enjoy or some pleasant experience. This is your time, just for these few minutes, no one or nothing else requires your attention. You may feel heat, cold or tingling from the Healer's hands. Most patients experience a feeling of peace and calm, relieved of tension and a possible easing of pain.

If this is Spiritual Healing, will I get any clairvoyant messages?

It is against the Healer's Code of Conduct to give clairvoyant messages. In any case pure Natural Healing comes from a slightly different source, consequently clairvoyant messages could interfere with the channelling of healing.

What safeguards have I got to ascertain if the Healer is properly trained?

Ask to see the Healer's current Membership Card. This card will show that the Healer is a current member of an Approved Association and that the Healer is fully insured. The Healer is thereby bound by a strict Code of Conduct

Now I am receiving healing, can I stop seeing my doctor?

Natural Healing is not alternative to, but complimentary to, any treatment prescribed by your doctor. The doctor is still in charge and you should carry on with your doctor's treatment. By all means tell your doctor that you are having Natural Healing.

Certain parts of the Code of Conduct refer specifically to Healer and Doctor relationships:-

1. A Healer must always ask whether you have consulted a doctor about your medical condition and formally advise you to do so if you have not.
2. A Healer is forbidden to countermand the advice or medical treatment prescribed by your doctor or to advise upon it.

This applies even more strenuously where a parent or guardian brings a child for healing.

Can you tell me what is wrong and what should I take?

Once again this is dealt with in the Code of Conduct, The Healer is forbidden to make a diagnosis, that is the prerogative of your doctor. Natural Healing is complimentary and non-invasive. We do not prescribe medicines of any kind. The benefits you derive from healing are completely natural.

Can healing help everyone?

It is most unusual for anyone not to receive some benefit from healing. You may begin to feel more confident, calmer with a little more get-up-and-go in your attitude. Healing can also have the effect of making you more tolerant of others.

Healing can help the terminally ill by easing of pain and giving a sense of peace and tranquillity. In some it helps to get rid of the fear of death.

The bereaved can also receive benefit from healing.

A Healer is forbidden by law to give healing to a woman in childbirth and for a period of ten days after.

Do I have to attend a Clinic for healing?

No, arrangements can be made for you to receive healing at home, if required. Healing sessions are often held at your local Spiritual Church, enquiries could be made there. The Alliance of Healing Associations comprises of around 25 Associations, with a total membership of 3,500 to 4,000 Healers. Enquiries can be made on the internet. One such contact would be:- www.surreyhealers.org.uk.

Can a child have healing?

Yes, with the permission of the parent or guardian. Here we must refer back to the relationship between Healer and Doctor. The law demands that a parent or guardian must seek qualified medical aid regarding the health of a child.

My dog isn't very well. Can he have healing?

Yes, on the understanding that the laying on of hands does not include the practise of Veterinary Surgery, but the Healer will always ask if the animal has been seen by a Veterinary Surgeon. In all instances where there is concern about the health of the animal the Healer must advise the owner to have the animal examined by a Veterinary Surgeon. The Veterinary Surgeon remains in charge of the case and the Healer must not countermand any instructions or medicines given by the Veterinary Surgeon.

As with Healer/Human patient relationship the Healer cannot make a diagnosis or advise a course of treatment.

CHAPTER 8

CODE OF CONDUCT

The Code of Conduct has been referred to several times within this book and therefore may need further explanation. Here I have listed a selection of the more salient points applicable to all Healers , who are members of an Approved Association.

Relationship with the Patient.

1. Healers should strive for excellence at all times, exemplifying the highest standards of professional behaviour and performance.
2. Healers must have respect for religious, spiritual, political and social views of any individual irrespective of race, colour, creed or sex and must never seek to impose their beliefs on a patient.

3. Healers must at all times conduct themselves in an honourable and courteous manner and with due diligence in their relations with their patients/clients and the public. They should seek a good relationship and shall work in a co-operative manner with other healthcare professionals and recognise and respect their particular contribution within the healthcare team, irrespective of whether they perform from an allopathic or alternative/complimentary base.

4. The relationship between healers and their patients/clients is that of a professional with a patient/ client. The patient places trust in the healer's care, skill and integrity and it is the healer's duty to act with due diligence at all times and not to abuse this trust in any way.

5. Proper moral conduct must always be paramount in a healers' relations with patients/clients. They must behave with courtesy, respect, dignity, discretion and tact. Their attitude must be competent and sympathetic, hopeful and positive, thus encouraging an uplift in the patient's mental outlook and belief in a progression towards good health practices.

6. Healers must never claim to 'cure'. The possible therapeutic benefits may be described, 'recovery' must never be guaranteed.

7. Healers must guard against the danger that a patient/client without previously consulting a Doctor may come for therapy for a known disorder and subsequently be found, too late, to be suffering from another serious disorder. To this end new patients/clients must be asked what medical advice they have received. If they have not seen a Doctor, they must be advised to do so. Since it is legal to refuse medical treatment, no patient/client can be forced to consult a Doctor. The advice must be recorded for the healer's protection and signed by the patient/client or their representative.

8. Healers must communicate clearly, effectively and openly to their patient/client.

9. Before giving treatment, healers must explain as fully as possible what will be involved in the treatment including the approximate length of treatment and fees, if appropriate.

10. Healers must act with consideration concerning fees.

11. Healers must not be judgmental and they should recognise the patient's/client's right to refuse treatment and to ignore advice. It is the patient's/client's prerogative to make their own choices with regard to their health, lifestyle and finances. By

the same token, the patient/client must recognise the healer's right to refuse treatment.

This section continues to include instructions regarding security of records, presence of third parties at healing sessions, healing of children and dealing with suspicion of child abuse.

Healer Awareness

1. Healers should continue to develop their knowledge and keep up to date with best practice.
2. Healers should ensure that they themselves are medically, physically and psychologically fit to practice.
3. Discretion must be used for the protection of the healer when carrying out private treatment with patients/clients who are mentally unstable, addicted to drugs or alcohol, or severely depressed suicidal or hallucinated. Such patients/clients must be treated by a healer (not a student) with relative competency, accompanied by another healer or practitioner. A healer must not treat a patient/client in any case which exceeds his capacity, training and competence. Where appropriate, the healer must seek referral to a more qualified person.

4. Healers are forbidden to diagnose, perform tests or treat animals in any way or give advice following diagnosis by a Registered Veterinary Surgeon or to countermand his instructions. (Excepting complementary treatment by the laying on of hands)

5. Healers must not apply contact healing to women in childbirth or treat them for ten days thereafter, (excluding distant or prayer healing).

6. Healers must not practise dentistry, even of they hold an appropriate qualification, whilst giving healing to a patient/client.

7. Healers must not charge a fee to, or accept a donation from, a patient suffering from a venereal disease as defined in the 1917 Act.

8. Patients suffering from Aids or other possible contagious diseases, may be treated at the discretion of the healer, who should take proper precautions of health and safety.

9. Healers must not use manipulation or massage while giving healing even if they possess an appropriate professional qualification.

10. Healers must not practise any other therapy, even if they hold an appropriate qualification, while giving healing to a patient/client.

11. Healers must not prescribe remedies, herbs, supplements, oils etc. If their training and

qualifications in another discipline entitles them to do so, practitioners may so prescribe, but not as part of the healing treatment they give.

12. Deals with the Data Protection Act

13. If a healer becomes aware that the patient/client is suffering from a Notifiable Disease, the patient must be advised to consult their Doctor as soon as possible. A list of these diseases is included in the Code.

These are followed by Sections on Administration and Publicity, Keeping of Records and Insurance and Guidelines for working with other Healthcare Professionals. Some of these important guidelines are:

1. Healers must not countermand instructions or prescriptions given by a Doctor.

2. Healers must not advise a particular course of medical treatment, such as to undergo an operation or take specific drugs. It must be left to the patient's/client's to make their own decision in the light of medical advice.

3. Healers must never give a medical diagnosis to a patient/client in any circumstances, this is the responsibility of a Registered Medical Practitioner.

Guidelines for working in Hospitals.

These cover the hospitals continued responsibility for the patient, the importance of gaining permission from hospital staff, not giving the impression of being a member of the hospital staff and the manner in which healing is provided.

This is followed by a short paragraph on Healing and the Law.

Next we have Additional Principals

1. Healers must never offer a clairvoyant reading during a healing session.
2. Explains trance healing.
3. Trance healing is forbidden for all members and is not included in the training programme.
4. Healers must consciously avoid saying or doing anything that contravenes the Code of Conduct.
5. Contact healing must only be given in response to an invitation from the patient or their representative.
6. To avoid offending some patients/clients healers must never raise the question of their religious beliefs unless this is invited by the patient/client.
7. When a healer is giving healing privately to a person of the opposite sex it is advisable for the healer to request the presence of a third party.

This is followed by ' Treatment of Animals' which gives additional rules for the healing of animals. These include, not diagnosing, the importance of advising the owner to seek Veterinary treatment, if deemed necessary, and healing only within the provisions of the Code.

Next Equal Opportunities Policies to deal with any forms of discrimination are listed. Finally there is a Section on Complaints and Disciplinary Procedures.

As can be seen the Code of Conduct, which must be adhered to, is a very comprehensive document.